Distribution, publication, and copying in any form are prohibited and subject to damages.

TEN HYPNOSES

Copying, publishing, and sharing with third parties are only permitted with the written consent of the author. Please observe the notes on copyright and usage.

Distribution, publication, and copying in any form are prohibited and subject to damages.

Copying, publishing, and sharing with third parties are only permitted with the written consent of the author. Please observe the notes on copyright and usage.

Distribution, publication, and copying in any form are prohibited and subject to damages.

Ingo Michael Simon

TEN HYPNOSES

43
BODY RELAXATION

Copying, publishing, and sharing with third parties are only permitted with the written consent of the author. Please observe the notes on copyright and usage.

© 2024 Ingo Michael Simon
All rights reserved.
Independently published
www.ingosimon.com

Important Notes for Urgent Attention:

The contents of this book are based on the practical experiences of the author with hypnosis applications and psychotherapy in a trance state. Although the author has strived for the utmost care, errors or misunderstandings in the presentation cannot be completely excluded. Therapeutic work with people and the application of hypnosis are solely the responsibility of the hypnotist. It cannot be ruled out that parts of this book may be misunderstood or that the application of a presented procedure may cause an undesirable reaction in the client. The author also assumes no co-responsibility if work with a client is carried out with reference to the statements in this book.

The Author:

Ingo Michael Simon studied psychology and education and is a hypnotherapist with practices in southwestern Germany and Switzerland. With the help of hypnosis-supported psychotherapy, he primarily treats people with persistent psychological conditions. His practice focuses on anxiety disorders, pathological compulsions, and psychosomatic illnesses. His therapeutic offerings mainly include classical and modern hypnosis applications and the dreamland therapy he developed himself.

Distribution, publication, and copying in any form are prohibited and subject to damages.

INTRODUCTION	6
COPYRIGHT AND USAGE	8
HYPNOSIS 1	10
HYPNOSIS 2	14
HYPNOSIS 3	19
HYPNOSIS 4	24
HYPNOSIS 5	30
HYPNOSIS 6	35
HYPNOSIS 7	40
HYPNOSIS 8	45
HYPNOSIS 9	50
HYPNOSIS 10	53
ALL TITLES IN THE SERIES	59

Copying, publishing, and sharing with third parties are only permitted with the written consent of the author. Please observe the notes on copyright and usage.

Introduction

The series "Ten Hypnoses" is very well known in Germany, Austria, and Switzerland as a collection of texts for therapeutic work and is used by numerous psychotherapeutic practices, doctors, therapists, coaches, and other helping professionals. I am pleased to now be able to offer these texts in other countries as well.

Most therapists have their own methods for inducing and deepening trance as well as for exiting trance. Therefore, I have focused on the main part of the hypnosis. The texts in this book can be integrated as the main part into any hypnosis process. The texts in this collection use various hypnosis techniques. I will not explain these in detail, as I assume that users have the appropriate training. It is also not necessary to understand the exact structure or functioning of the different parts. The texts can simply be read aloud, and they will have their effect.

Decide for yourself which text best suits your client or patient at any given time. You can also combine passages from different texts. It is not about using all ten hypnoses in sequence. It is a selection of possibilities.

I want to emphasize that books cannot replace therapy. Psychotherapy or other therapeutic treatments involve much more. A careful diagnosis is the necessary basis for deciding on the use of methods, including whether hypnosis or one of my texts should be used. Even in this case, preparatory discussions, follow-up discussions during the session, and of course, a therapeutic concept for the sequence of sessions and the content approaches are essential parts of therapy. This cannot and should not be achieved with a collection of texts.

In any case, I wish you much success in your work and I am pleased if my text templates can contribute in a small way.

Ingo Michael Simon

Copyright and Usage

Copying, publishing, and sharing with third parties is prohibited and only permitted with the written consent of the author. Please observe the following copyright and usage guidelines.

This work has been carefully crafted and created to the best of the author's knowledge and personal experience. It comprises text templates and application guidelines for professional hypnosis sessions. The author is a licensed psychotherapist with extensive experience in psychotherapy, coaching, and personal training using hypnotic techniques and methods. Nevertheless, the author and the publisher assume no liability for the accuracy of information, instructions, and advice, nor for any typographical errors. The author and publisher accept no responsibility or liability for the application of these texts and recommendations with clients or patients, nor for any potential consequences or unexpected reactions. It is expressly noted that the application of therapeutic and advisory techniques and formulations lies solely and entirely within the responsibility of the practitioner. This also applies to adherence to the boundaries of legally regulated medical and therapeutic practices. The fact that a book containing action proposals is freely available for sale does not imply that its application with clients or patients is permitted for everyone.

Hypnosis 1

... ... Today, you will find your way into a truly deep and very healing physical relaxation ... ... Physically relaxing often seems simple because when you lie down and rest, your body naturally relaxes ... ... This happens automatically as you move less ... ... But what you need is a much deeper ... ... a much more intense relaxation of the body ... ... Perhaps there are tensions or tightness in your muscles ... ... or aching or strained tendons and ligaments ... ... or joints that have become weak points in your body due to the stresses of daily life, work, or sports ... ... Just as we sometimes need a mental and emotional break to truly unwind, our body also needs a break to relax deeply ... ... Your body needs this break ... ... and you are giving it to yourself now ... ... You are giving yourself a true and healing break for your body in this trance ... ... This hypnosis is your wellness vacation ... ... Perhaps you knew that in hypnosis, you can experience and achieve more in a very short time than in a waking state ... ... because in hypnosis, there is no time ... ... It often feels like a long, restful time has passed, even though only a few minutes have gone by ... ... That is the great advantage of hypnosis ... ... Everything happens in peace, but much faster than you are used to ... ... So let's begin and take care of your healing physical relaxation together ... ...

... ... Perhaps you have wondered how we will start ... ... or you have already noticed that we have been at it for minutes, and that your healing physical relaxation has already begun ... ... You are already guiding your body into this restful and peaceful state of relaxation ... ... and with every word you hear, you take your body further down this path of healing relaxation ... ... the path of recovery and regeneration ... ... You don't need to do anything special for this ... ... Once you have reached the point of physical trance, you only need to feel the relaxation of your body in your thoughts and feelings ... ... And perhaps you have noticed that you have already reached the point of physical trance ... ... Your body has already entered this state of trance and can find ever deeper rest there ... ... Maybe you are wondering what a physical trance actually is ... ... But why ask ... ... when you can experience it now ... ... when you can feel it now ... ... This special relaxation ... ... this letting go of your muscles ... ... This relief in your joints ... ... this tiredness and this freedom ... ... This is your physical trance, which is so healing ... ... Just follow the feeling of peace ... ... Just follow the feeling of your body ... ... good ... ... You can do it ... ...

... ... You feel your body ... ... Your body finds more and more peace and relief ... ... relaxes and relaxes ... ... and wherever there may be tensions or pain, this peace now also sets in ... ... this healing peace ... ... Step by step, you feel the relaxation of your body more clearly and feel the good feeling that spreads with it ... ... a sense of well-being that permeates your body ... ... and if you find a spot that is not yet relaxed and comfortable, then let the peace of your muscles and the peace of all the already relaxed parts of your body flow there ... ... so that your body is increasingly embraced by the healing peace and all tensions fade away ... ... Your body finds the depth of trance ... ... now ... ... Your body feels good ... ... now ... ...

... ... You also feel freer in your mood than you did a few minutes ago ... ... because with the relaxation of your body ... ... with this healing and pleasant feeling, worries and fears fall away from you because now everything is okay ...

... Now is the time for deep rest ... ... Now is the time for inner peace ... ... Now is the time for a good feeling in your body ... ... Now is the time to be free from all burdens ... ... Free from all pain and only peace remains ... ... deep peace ... ... You feel free and light now ... ... You feel truly free and light now ... ... {about 20 seconds pause} ... ...

... ... Enjoy this state of deep and healing relaxation ... ... Realize that your body could relax faster and deeper than you expected ... ... But most importantly, realize that your body can always find this deep peace and relaxation again ... ... but only together with your thoughts and your feelings ... ... When you grant your body peace and follow it mindfully with your thoughts and feelings as you did today, you can always experience a very deep and especially healing relaxation of your body ... ... just like in this trance ... ... just like with this hypnosis ... ... Now continue to enjoy the relaxation ... ... and trust that the healing effect of this relaxation will continue to unfold even when you are back in your waking daily life ... ...

Hypnosis 2

...... You want to relax ...... You want and can now find a deep physical peace and relax and rejuvenate your body ... ... It is good and important that after a time of stress and exertion, we make sure to give our bodies enough care and attention so they can recover well and stay healthy ...... or, if they are already weakened or even sick, regain health, vitality, and strength ...... To do this, you turn your gaze inward and enter into a direct inner dialogue with your body ...... This dialogue takes place in your thoughts and in your feelings ...... Let the voice you hear become your inner voice so that your deep inner self, your subconscious, can absorb all the words ...... and your subconscious then directs the best words of relaxation directly to your body ... ... to every single cell, so that your body can experience optimal peace and relaxation ...... and ideal recovery ......

...... Start by relieving your body, which now only needs to feel itself ...... You know that every feeling also influences your body, and many stressful feelings could have additionally burdened your body ...... Now you turn inward and allow your body to be there only for itself and to relax ... ... With mindfulness and gratitude, you turn to your inner self and your entire body and assure it that you appreciate how often and how long it has worked well for you and functioned ... ... Then you say ...

... Now, dear body, I allow you to rest and recover ... ... Let go of all emotions and just be there for yourself ... ... Find deep peace and recovery ... ... Now ... ...

And then you feel into your body and sense that it has absorbed your words and is implementing them for its own recovery ... ... And as your body finds ever deeper peace, you think about what might help achieve an even deeper and more restful peace ... ... you think about the individual parts of your body that have worked so well and carried so many burdens ... ... and you turn to each one with gratitude and recognition for every healthy moment of your life ... ... for every task your body has already done for you and with you ... ... So you say ... ... Dear head, you who coordinate all parts of the body, rest now because you have earned it ... {about 5 seconds pause} ... and then you feel your head relaxing ever deeper ... ... Then you turn to your shoulders, knowing their contribution, and say ... ... Dear shoulders, I want you to rest and recover now because you have always held the arms and hands when they seemed to be working alone ... {about 5 seconds pause} ...

... ... and then you feel your shoulders loosening and deeply relaxing ... ... And similarly, you turn to your arms and hands, which are so often in motion every day ... ... You want them to find deep peace as well, and you say ... ... Dear hands and arms, who do the work of holding and carrying ... ... Now you may let go ... ... Now there is nothing to carry and nothing to hold ... ... Now is only a time of rest ... {about 5 seconds pause} ... ...

... ... and then you feel your arms and hands also relaxing and recovering ever deeper ... ... Then there is your upper body with all its organs, working unseen, which can also benefit from deep peace and deeply relax ... ... You know that these parts of your body also seek and can find peace when you turn to them with mindfulness ... ... So you also speak to these parts of your body and say ... ... Dear upper body and all you faithful organs within ... ... I know how valuable you are and how valuable your contribution is to a functioning whole ... ... so you too should rest and relax ... ... I want my entire upper body to deeply and thoroughly relax so that my body experiences a truly deep and very restful peace ... ... now ... {about 5 seconds pause} ... and then you feel your upper body relaxing ever deeper ... ... And finally, you turn mindfully to your legs and feet ... ... They carry you all day long, step by step, for you and with you ... ... You say to them ... ... Now allow yourselves to rest and relax, dear legs and feet ... ... I know that you carry the entire body every day, but now is truly a time of rest for you ... ... deep rest for you ... {about 5 seconds pause} ... ...

... ... and then you feel your legs and feet relaxing ever deeper ... ... Then you enjoy the peace together with your body, which you also feel in your thoughts and feelings ... ... Your entire being rests and relaxes ... ... And as your body, in particular, finds ever deeper peace and relaxes more and more, you think about how you can always find deep peace with mindfulness and attention to yourself, and will ... ... Perhaps you resolve to create a short and contemplative time of external and internal peace every day by lying down in peace and turning inward ... ... with mindfulness and with the conscious permission to relax ... ... just like today ... ... just as you are experiencing it now ... ... and each day you find yourself more quickly in a truly restful state of inner peace ... ...

Hypnosis 3

... ... Today, you are experiencing a truly deep relaxation ... for an intensive recovery of your body ... ... and this relaxation happens very quickly ... ...

... ... Today, you are experiencing a truly deep relaxation ... for an intensive recovery of your body ... ... and this relaxation is restorative and refreshing ... ...

... ... Today, you are experiencing a truly deep relaxation ... for an intensive recovery of your body ... ... and in doing so, your body finds a truly deep peace ... ...

... ... Today, you are experiencing a truly deep relaxation ... for an intensive recovery of your body ... ... because you let all the words flow gently and calmly into your inner self ... ...

... ... To do this, let go of all thoughts now ... let them drift away like clouds in the sky ... ... and you become free and open to a truly deep peace ... ...

... ... To do this, let go of all thoughts now ... let them drift away like clouds in the sky ... ... and with the letting go of thoughts, your body relaxes even deeper ... ...

... ... To do this, let go of all thoughts now ... let them drift away like clouds in the sky ... ... and your muscles and tendons let go as well ... ...

... ... To do this, let go of all thoughts now ... let them drift away like clouds in the sky ... ... and all the tensions in your body dissolve ... ...

... ... Your body becomes increasingly calm, all muscles and tendons let go ... ... Now ... ...

... ... With every exhale, it gets quieter within you and your body becomes tired ... ... and your body feels as good as in a deep sleep ... ...

... ... With every exhale, it gets quieter within you and your body becomes tired ... ... and with that, you already feel the recovery of your body in the peace ... ...

... ... With every exhale, it gets quieter within you and your body becomes tired ... ... and as in sleep, the muscles and tendons become even looser ... ...

... ... With every exhale, it gets quieter within you and your body becomes tired ... ... and all muscles and tendons are flexible like rubber ... ...

... ... Your body becomes increasingly calm, all muscles and tendons let go ... ... Now ... ...

... ... You are filled with a deep sense of inner freedom and peace ... ... and this peace spreads throughout your body ...

... ... You are filled with a deep sense of inner freedom and peace ... ... and this peace also creates a comfortable feeling in your body ... ...

... ... You are filled with a deep sense of inner freedom and peace ... ... and this state feels like a beautiful dream ... ...

... ... You are filled with a deep sense of inner freedom and peace ... ... and in this peace, you can let go of everything that could still bother you ... ...

... ... Your body becomes increasingly calm, all muscles and tendons let go ... ... Now ... ...

… … Now, you don't have to do anything yourself … You can just enjoy the peace … … … because in this deep relaxation, everything happens on its own … …

… … Now, you don't have to do anything yourself … You can just enjoy the peace … … … because only when you do nothing now can your body truly relax deeply … …

… … Now, you don't have to do anything yourself … You can just enjoy the peace … … … because in doing so, you feel that your body is indeed resting deeply now … …

… … Now, you don't have to do anything yourself … You can just enjoy the peace … … … because deep peace is what you deserve, and deep peace is what your body deserves … .

… … Your body becomes increasingly calm, all muscles and tendons let go … … Now … …

… … Now feel the deep peace of the trance and feel your body, which is as relaxed as it hasn't been for a long time … … and you can always reach this relaxation again in peace …

… … Now feel the deep peace of the trance and feel your body, which is as relaxed as it hasn't been for a long time … … and this relaxation gives your body new strength … …

… … Now feel the deep peace of the trance and feel your body, which is as relaxed as it hasn't been for a long time … … and in this relaxation, every cell of your body regenerates … …

… … Feel and enjoy the deep peace of the trance … … Feel and enjoy the peace in your body … …

Hypnosis 4

... ... You want to achieve a very special relaxation of your body today ... ... a truly deep relaxation because you know that the body sometimes only seems to rest ... ... When you lie still, it initially appears that your body is already completely relaxed and loose ... ... But then you notice, if you really pay attention, that your body can relax much more deeply ... ... that it can truly let go much more ... ... and you have chosen this hypnosis because you want to finally experience this even deeper relaxation ... ... because you really want to feel a deep physical peace ... ... with the relief of all muscles and joints ... ... with the relief of the body parts that so often bear the burdens of everyday life ... ... So now it is also important to relax your feet, and this is easy ... ... because normally they carry the weight of your body all day long ... ... Now it's different, now even your feet can find rest ... ... and your shoulders ... ... They are involved in every movement of lifting and carrying, constantly in motion ... ... but now it's different ... ... now even your shoulders can rest ... ... and your hands ... ...

because your hands do most of the work during the day ... ... but now it's different ... ... Now it is also possible for your hands to relax ... ... and as you think about this, you realize that many parts of your body are constantly in motion or at work ... ...

... ... But in everyday life, it often doesn't seem that way to you ... ... and you don't notice how much work your body does because you're used to it ... ... But now you have time for yourself ... ... Time for yourself and for your body ... ... So now let your breath flow calmly and notice how it flows in and out ... ... You can feel the breath at the wings of your nose ... ... It feels a bit cool when you breathe in ... ... and a bit warmer when you breathe out ... ... and you can also observe the path of the air in your body ... ... You feel how your breath flows through your nose and throat into your lungs ... ... and you can imagine it ... ... as if you were taking a journey through your body with the air you breathe ... ... through your nose ... ... down the airways ... ... to the lungs ... ... and back again ... ... But you can imagine more than that ... ... You can imagine that you could breathe into your entire body ... ... that you can direct your breath ... ... into the lungs and beyond ... ... initially as an idea, as a fantasy ... ... But then you will quickly feel and experience that exactly this idea of the breath flowing into your entire body leads to a very deep relaxation ... ... can even dissolve tension or pain ... ... Imagine directing the air with your next breath to where your body really needs to relax ... ...

... ... So now breathe into your shoulders ... ... Breathe in and guide your breath through your nose to your shoulders and into your arms ... ... Your breath finds a smooth and harmonious path into your arms, which relax as it flows ... ... It flows all the way to your hands and fingertips ... ... and your hands and fingers also come to rest ... ... and harmoniously, the air flows back through your nose as you exhale, leaving your body ... ... and your shoulders are relaxed ... ... your arms are relaxed ... ... your hands are relaxed ... ... But maybe you also have the feeling that the air is getting stuck or swirling around, not flowing as harmoniously ... ... If that's the case, it just shows you that your shoulders and arms can and want to relax even more deeply ... ... Then direct your breath with the next inhalations precisely to where you feel the swirling or blockage ... ... and then that spot relaxes ... ... then you feel the healing and soothing effect exactly there ... ... Breathe for your peace ... ... Breathe for your body ... ... Breathe for your relaxation ... ... {about 5-10 seconds pause} ... ...

... ... Your body has understood and continues to breathe for you into your shoulders and arms as you move on ... ... and your shoulders and arms become more and more peaceful ... ... and your hands too ... ... Likewise, now breathe into your upper body ... ... into the lungs and beyond into the abdominal area ... ... to all the internal organs ... ... Your breath finds a harmonious path through your upper body ... ... through the abdominal area and perhaps through the spine back to your nose ... ... who knows ... ... You find the best path ... ... You find the path that allows your body to relax the most ... ... and if there's a spot that bothers or burdens you in some way, you know what to do ... ... Direct your breath there ... ... then you feel the healing and soothing effect exactly there ... ... And if you have the feeling or impression that your breath is getting stuck somewhere or taking a detour because something is bothering you, then breathe exactly there ... ... Direct your breath exactly to where something might bother or burden you ... ... then you will feel the healing and soothing effect there too, and your breath will find the harmonious path again ... ... Breathe for your peace ... ... Breathe for your body ... ... Breathe for your relaxation ... ... {about 5-10 seconds pause} ... ...

... ... Your body has also taken this in and continues to breathe for the relaxation of your upper body ... ... Relaxation of the abdomen ... ... Relaxation of the back ... ... good ... ... your body finds ever deeper peace, and it goes as if guided by a magical hand ... ... because you can control your breath, and your body gladly follows this idea ... ... for a truly deep relaxation ... ... for deep inner peace that you can feel more and more intensely ... ... Finally, move on to your legs and feet, because they too need relief and rest ... ... Direct your breath with the next inhalations down into your legs and let it flow all the way into your feet ... ... And in your legs and feet, the same thing happens ... ... With the harmonious flow of breath into the legs and feet and back to your nose, your legs and feet finally come to rest and find the deep relaxation that your entire body has now already reached ... ... Let your breath flow evenly, and if anything could distract it, you know what to do ... ... Breathe exactly there and find harmony and deep relaxation ... ... Breathe for your peace ... ... Breathe for your body ... ... Breathe for your relaxation ... ... {about 10-15 seconds pause} ... ...

... ... Your body has reached a very deep relaxation ... ... All muscles and tendons are finding regeneration and recovery ... ... All joints are finding new strength in this beautiful peace ... ... Your body enjoys this deep peace with you and draws new strength and vitality for the day from it ... ... And you know that you can always breathe for the relaxation of your body ... ... conscious breathing helps you relax and rest at any time ... ... just like here and today ... ... just like here and today ... ...

Hypnosis 5

... ... Now you want to experience a very deep relaxation ... ... a relaxation that is good for your body and also allows your thoughts and mood to rest ... ... an inner peace, then ... ... an inner peace that lets you relax more deeply than a very restful sleep ... ... That is possible because you have already reached a special state of relaxation ... ... You are in a trance ... ... and perhaps this trance feels very ordinary to you ... ... like the moment just before a nap ... ... and indeed, trance is similar, but it is also different in a special way ... ... because while you can still perceive your surroundings, unlike in sleep, and hear my words, deep inside very special things are happening ... ... For example, it is possible for your body to rest and relax deeply inside while you only perceive the external relaxation of your body, the peace of the muscles and the movement system ... ... But your body can relax much more deeply, and it is already doing so ... ... and you can help your body ...

... ... When you are in a trance, images and inner pictures become friendly prompts and aids for your subconscious and for your body, which behave like the pictures you imagine ... ... Perhaps you knew this because you are familiar with hypnosis or because you have informed yourself about how and why it works ... ... or you are surprised and interested to hear and experience that it actually works and functions exactly this way ... ... You want to experience a beautiful and deep physical peace, so imagine that there are small clouds of tension in your body ... ... They are like clouds in the sky ... ... No one can stop them when they start to move, just as no one can stop the clouds in the sky ... ... not even you ... ... And your breath is like the wind high up in the sky, driving the clouds and even dissolving them when it blows ... ... In still air, the clouds remain stationary, and so too would the clouds of tension in you remain stationary ... ... But your breath is like the wind ... ... Your inhaling and exhaling is the wind that can move and dissolve the clouds of tension in your body ... ... and this wind never stands still unless you were to hold your breath ... ... But why would you do that? ... ... You want to feel good, and above all ... ... You want to relax ... ... So you breathe calmly and evenly ... ... So the wind of your breath blows through your body ... ... and it finds and moves the clouds of tension ... ... dissolves them ... ... The clearer you can imagine small clouds of tension in your body and the better you can imagine your breath as wind, the faster your body reacts to it and actually dissolves the tensions ... ... and your body finds deep peace ... ... You hear the sound of your breath ... ... You hear the inhaling and the exhaling ... ... and that's why it is really easy to imagine all this ... ... because then relaxation happens by itself ... ... then it is no longer possible not to find a very deep peace ...

... ... So let the wind of your breath blow through your body ... ... into every corner of your body, the wind of your breath flows and drives the clouds of tension together ... ... Everywhere small clouds of tension move through your body, and it feels good that they start to move ... ... because with each cloud ... ... with each tension that dissolves and moves, your body already becomes calmer and relaxes more deeply ... ... deeper and deeper ... ... From all the corners and crevices of your body, tension clouds dissolve and are driven by the wind of your breath to the center of your body and gather there in all peace ... ... in the center ... ... where the gut feeling is ... ... You feel the wind of your breath flowing through your body ... ... searching for tension clouds that it finds and dissolves ... ... They move with a good feeling to the center of your body and gather there as a thick, white cloud, which already feels light and soft ... ... Imagine it just like that ... ... Let this inner image of white clouds emerge ... ... of small tension clouds that dissolve everywhere in your body and move to the center of your body, driven by the wind of your breath, which constantly flows through your whole body ... ... So slowly, all tensions flow gently and lightly to the center of your body ... ... so gently and so lightly that you hardly feel them anymore, and your whole body relaxes deeply ... ... sinks into a very deep trance and experiences a wonderful state of peace there ... ... And now all the tensions arrive in the center of your body ... ... Every tension in your body that might still be there dissolves and gathers in the large white cloud in the center of your body ... ... good ... ... That's good ... ... In a few moments, you will experience an even deeper relaxation ... ... {about 10 seconds pause} ...

... ... Because now you are only breathing into the center of your body, to completely dissolve all tensions ... ... Your breath flows into the center of your body and dissolves the cloud of tensions there like a warm spring wind dissolves clouds in the sky ... ... You are only breathing toward your body's center now ... ... There your breath dissolves every tension completely ... ... You feel the relaxation of your body with every breath ... ... Every breath lets your body relax more deeply ... ... now ... ... {about 20 seconds pause} ...

... ... Now you can let go of the image of the clouds because they have already completely dissolved ... ... and your body has found a deep peace ... ... a peace and a real relaxation that goes much deeper than your immediate perception ... ... But maybe you can feel it after all, if you dive deep into your feeling ... ... Then you feel the deep relaxation of your body ... ... deep relaxation ... ...

Hypnosis 6

... ... You now want to experience a truly deep physical relaxation as quickly as possible ... ... and with the relaxation of your body also a beautiful inner peace ... ... The relaxation you already feel helps you with this ... ... but it is only an important first step ... ... And as the next step, you can experience an even deeper and more pleasant relaxation ... ... That's very simple ... ... I will show you the way there ... ... Just calmly follow my voice, which guides you and shows you this simple and highly effective path into the depths of relaxation ... ... Just enjoy the peace ... ... and fully immerse yourself in the feeling of deep relaxation ... ... Now ... ...

... ... Perhaps you know that a mindful turning toward yourself leads to a genuine and very deep peace when you want to rest ... ... to a peace that also encompasses your entire body like a pleasant fatigue in the evening that draws you into sleep so that you can fully rest and recover ... ... Mindful turning toward yourself can be shaped by a thought of self-care and the inner permission you give yourself ... ...

with a permission that you grant yourself ... ... very consciously and with full conviction because this allows your inner self, your subconscious, to truly believe and accept your permission ... ... and immediately lead your body into a very calm state ... ... into a state of complete well-being ... ... So you need a formulation for your mindful turning toward yourself ... ... an affirmation ... ... An affirmation is like a formula that helps you today to achieve deep physical peace ... ... and it helps you again and again to achieve this physical peace ... ...

... ... Today, you can guide your body into a state of genuine and deep relaxation with the affirmation ... ... simply by hearing the affirmation and adopting it as your own attitude ... ... This is very simple because its content aligns with your desire for peace ... ... and when you are fully awake again and back in your daily life, you can always use this affirmation yourself whenever you seek a moment of mindfulness and inner reflection ... ... And as soon as you do this, your body will strive for a very restorative state of relaxation ...

... ... Now feel your body sensation ... ... Let the peace you already feel work ... ... It has a calming effect on your thoughts and your body and helps you to relax both your thoughts and your body ... ... and you can use physical relaxation very well now ... ... because now you especially want to do something good for your body ... ... and really help your body deeply relax now ... ... So you take the following words deep within you as if they were your own words ... ... You make them your words because they align with your desire for peace ... ... You hear and say inside ... {5-10 seconds pause} ...

... ... I open myself to the silence deep within me and enjoy the peace, and I allow my body to let go and rest with me ... ...

... {Read the affirmations slightly slower and louder than the rest of the text, and pause for 5-10 seconds after each affirmation before continuing to read!} ...

... ... And now simply feel the peace because this allows the heard affirmation to best become your inner attitude ... ... Feel the peace and the genuine relaxation of your body and sense how your affirmation actually allows your body to relax more deeply ... ... You certainly feel it already ... ... or you will feel it even more clearly in a few moments and sink with your body into a very deep peace that is as restful as many hours of sleep ... ... many restful hours of sleep in just a few moments ... ...

... ... Perhaps your affirmation was just a good intention or a statement of intent a short time ago, but in this trance, it has become your inner attitude ... ... a constructive attitude that causes deep physical relaxation ... ... You feel this affirmation, it echoes within you like an echo ... ...

... ... I open myself to the silence deep within me and enjoy the peace, and I allow my body to let go and rest with me ... ...

... {Read the affirmations slightly slower and louder than the rest of the text, and pause for 5-10 seconds after each affirmation before continuing to read!} ...

... ... Allow this echo to unfold its relaxing and calming effect ... ... Your body has already responded clearly to the affirmation because your body has found peace and recovery ... ... and the heard affirmation has become your very own peace affirmation ... ... Whenever you seek peace and physical relaxation, you can make yourself comfortable, just like now ... ... then close your eyes and whisper your affirmation, which immediately leads you into a state of physical peace ... ... into a state of physical peace and recovery ... ... just like now ... ...

Hypnosis 7

... ... With this hypnosis, you can experience a state of deep physical peace ... ... It's very simple and completely safe ... ... You don't need to do much for it ... ... You just need to listen, that's enough ... ... Yes, it is absolutely enough to listen ... ... to listen and take in the words you hear ... ... Your subconscious examines every word you hear carefully ... ... You can rely on that ... ... because your subconscious knows very well that there are helpful words ... ... Formulations that make it easier for you to experience a truly deep peace and relaxation of your body ... ... Strictly speaking, you can relax without any words ... ... very deeply relax ... ... Every person can experience a state of deep physical relaxation ... ... so can you ... ... We can all do it when our thoughts come to rest ... ... But it is not always easy to let your thoughts rest ... ... But that's exactly what this hypnosis is for ... ... While you can let your thoughts wander or take a mental journey ... ... think about one thing or another that comes to mind ... ... your subconscious simply listens ... ... Your subconscious always hears all the words I speak for you ... ... So you have a free choice to listen as well ... ... or simply go your own way in your thoughts and trust your subconscious ...

... ... Surely you have already experienced very intense physical relaxation ... ... maybe in sleep or in meditation ... ... Even if it might not be easy for you right now to achieve such relaxation or if it hasn't been so easy lately, you do know what the state of truly deep and restorative physical peace feels like ... ... And because you know this and have already experienced it, your body can also reach such a state today ... ... Your body is now striving for the state of deep relaxation, and you can already feel it ... ... And indeed, it is now possible for you to relax more and more deeply and also to feel and enjoy this ever-deepening physical peace ... ... Enjoy the peace you feel and let yourself sink deeper and deeper into this peace ... ... You are in complete safety and can let yourself sink into the deep peace ... ... Enjoy this relaxation because now is a time just for you ... ... just for you and for the rest and recovery of your body ... ... That's right ... ... That's good ... ... Your subconscious helps you ... ... Your subconscious carries you safely into the depths of relaxation and ever deeper into inner peace ... ... and your body relaxes more and more ... ... All muscles let go ... ... All muscles and all tendons finally let go ... ... Now ... ...

... ... You can let your thoughts wander and simply let individual thoughts come and go ... ... But maybe it's already the case that your thoughts no longer interest you because you only want to perceive your feeling ... ... Feel into your feelings, your emotions, and moods ... ... All thoughts become unimportant ... ... Now, only your feeling counts ... ... Now, only your feeling counts ... ... and you feel peace ... ... You feel the peace of your body ... ... You connect the feeling and sensing with the deep inner peace and let all thoughts that might arise simply pass by ... ... You increasingly feel that it's only about the feeling because when you immerse yourself in the feeling, your body relaxes best ... ... by letting go of thoughts, your body already sinks into a truly deep and genuine relaxation and recovery ... ... Relaxation can be that simple ... ... Relaxation is that simple ... ... and you can reach it again and again whenever you want to experience it ... ... You simply let your thoughts wander ... ... and your body relaxes very deeply ... ... You simply let all thoughts pass by ... ... Every thought that might arise, you immediately let pass by ... ... and your body relaxes very deeply ... ... You completely immerse yourself in your feeling ... ... and your body experiences a very pleasant relaxation ... ... very pleasant ... ... just like now ... ...

... ... Now enjoy the peace and relaxation completely ... ... Your body has arrived in a deep peace ... ... You can, of course, move and, if you like, lie down even more comfortably ... ... Now use the time to consciously feel the peace and benefit twice ... ... on the one hand for even more pleasant physical relaxation ... ... on the other hand for the enjoyable doing nothing and inner rest ... ... Now feel the relaxation and consciously perceive it ... ... Let the feeling of peace take up more and more space and immerse yourself more and more in this outer and inner peace ... ... Now nothing else is important but only your outer and inner peace ... ... only your outer and inner peace ... ... and the wonderful recovery that happens during this time ... ... That's good ... ... that feels good ... ... You can always experience this peace again ... ... simply by turning mindfully toward yourself ... ... by letting go and feeling ... ... This wonderful peace you can always enjoy and reach faster and faster because your inner self now knows the way there ...

... And this relaxation leads to a very special recovery ... ... to new strength and vitality that you feel immediately when you are awake again and move actively ... ... Today's relaxation and recovery is a complete success ... ...

Hypnosis 8

...... You focus internally on your goal of deep physical relaxation ...... because this way your body can truly relax and recover ...

...... At the same time, you are open to the words that accompany you on this path ...... because this way your body can truly relax and recover ...

...... You turn your mindful attention to your body sensation ...... because this way your body can truly relax and recover ...

...... And just as mindfully and attentively, you follow the helpful words that accompany you ...... because this way your body can truly relax and recover ...

...... You now simply let go of all strenuous thoughts ...... and with this thought, you also feel the ever-deepening peace of your body ...

...... You now only keep the thought of deep relaxation ...... and with this thought, you also feel the ever-deepening peace of your body ...

...... You focus entirely on the thought of peace ...... and with this thought, you also feel the ever-deepening peace of your body ...

...... Thus, the thought simply becomes a feeling of peace ...... and with this thought, you also feel the ever-deepening peace of your body ...

...... Deep peace spreads through your body ...... deep peace ...

...... You feel your body and become fully aware of it now ...... and this mindfulness allows your body to rest very deeply and securely ...

...... With this hypnosis, you give your body a time of peace and recovery ...... and this mindfulness allows your body to rest very deeply and securely ...

...... You breathe calmly and evenly for an even better body sensation ...... and this mindfulness allows your body to rest very deeply and securely ...

... ... You experience and consciously feel every little relaxation of your body ... ... and this mindfulness allows your body to rest very deeply and securely ...

... ... Deep peace spreads through your body ... ... deep peace ...

... ... You now let go of all disturbing thoughts ... ... with joy, you help your body perhaps the most in its deep and restful peace ...

... ... You rejoice in the feeling of peace and relaxation ... ... with joy, you help your body perhaps the most in its deep and restful peace ...

... ... You rejoice in this time-out for your body ... ... with joy, you help your body perhaps the most in its deep and restful peace ...

... ... You rejoice in this physical well-being ... ... with joy, you help your body perhaps the most in its deep and restful peace ...

... ... Deep peace spreads through your body ... ... deep peace ...

… … Just as now, you can always treat yourself and your body … … because this way, you give your body an appropriate recovery time again and again …

… … Every day you can create a time of peace and rest … … because this way, you give your body an appropriate recovery time again and again …

… … You are worth treating yourself with care again and again … … because this way, you give your body an appropriate recovery time again and again …

… … You are worth doing what helps you relax and find new strength … … because this way, you give your body an appropriate recovery time again and again …

… … Deep peace spreads through your body … … deep peace …

… … Today, you have attentively followed the helpful words … … and that is why your body has found a very restful peace and continues to recover …

… … You have understood and accepted the helpful words … … and that is why your body has found a very restful peace and continues to recover …

... ... The helpful words can therefore flow even deeper into your inner self ... ... and that is why your body has found a very restful peace and continues to recover ...

... ... You have walked an attentive path of peace and continue to walk it ... ... and that is why your body has found a very restful peace and continues to recover ...

Hypnosis 9

... ... After you have already found some peace and relaxation and have made yourself as comfortable as possible, you have so far managed well to attentively follow my words because you can hear my voice clearly and distinctly ... ... and your body relaxes more and more deeply ...

... ... You can perceive your surroundings with your senses even during hypnosis, feel, for example, that your body is being held stable by the surface that supports it, also hear the melody of the music playing in the background ... ... while you turn your gaze more and more inward and perceive your body, which releases all tensions and relaxes more deeply ...

... ... With your eyes closed, you still see light or color dots, that's normal ... ... and you also feel your breath flowing in and out at your nostrils ... ... And you can also feel and sense that your muscles are becoming looser, feel the relaxation of your tendons and ligaments, and you feel the peace of your joints, which are now relieved ...

... ... Every perception that interests you can become clear in trance, just like my voice, while you can always decide where to direct your attention, and of course, you can always recognize what helps you because you can check every helpful effect yourself to see if it serves your goal, or you simply trust completely if you are sure that everything is happening for your best ... ... and then you also trust in a truly deep relaxation of your body ...

... ... It's easy for you to concentrate on individual body parts or reactions, for example, you feel your breath very well when you pay attention to it, and you can feel and trace every breath exactly, and you can even count the next five breaths ... {one breath pause to allow the client to start counting inwardly and be slightly distracted} ... ... This way, tensions and even hardenings of your body are dissolved, and also possible feelings of pressure and pain are now really significantly reduced ...

... ... You feel your body, and you feel your surroundings ... You can perceive the external and also the internal, your emotions ... ... and your body reaches an ever deeper state of peace ... and a sense of well-being spreads, which even ends pressure and pain ...

… … Of course, you feel how far your body has relaxed because you are mindful of yourself, and therefore, you can also feel when the physical peace is so deep that you can clearly feel the recovery, and as soon as this deep state of relaxation has occurred, and you feel that you are already deeply relaxed … … … you also clearly feel that your body is more deeply relaxed than ever before and that all muscles are really loosened, that hardenings and feelings of pressure have actually completely dissolved and a good feeling has set in, and that your body finds in exactly this beautiful and deep peace a very healing recovery and new strength and vitality for the day …

Hypnosis 10

... ... You are looking for and finding deep relaxation of your body today ... ... a deeper peace and relaxation of your body than you might expect ... ... because in this beautiful peace trance, your body can relax down to the level of every single cell ... ... First, you feel the relief of the joints and muscles ... ... then the muscular relaxation and loosening ... ... and if you are very mindful and attentive to your innermost self, you may even be able to feel the very deep relaxation ... ... the relaxation that goes down to every body cell ... ... But you can let all this come to you in peace ... ... You don't need to do anything other than follow my voice a little and pay attention to the helpful words that promote relaxation ... ... On their own, you recognize them and hear them without any effort ... ... because helpful words somehow sound familiar because they are similar to your thoughts ... ... These are the words that work best ... ... But you don't have to actively find them, your subconscious finds them and accepts these words ...

... You have already found some peace and ... relaxation ...

... You have made yourself comfortable ...

... It ... succeeds ... in attentively following my words ...

... You hear these words clearly and ... distinctly ...

... And your body relaxes ... deeper and deeper ... relaxed ...

... Your senses function ... perfectly ...

... You feel your body with your senses ...

... The music in the background accompanies ... your trance ...

... Your gaze turns more and more ... inward ...

... And your body now releases all tensions ...

... Even with your eyes closed, your vision is ... intact ... {understood: in rhythm} ...

... Your skin feels every breath of air, even that ... of your breath ...

... And likewise, you can feel your muscles becoming ... looser ...

... You now also feel the ... relaxation ... of your tendons and ligaments ...

... You now also feel the ... relief ... of your joints ...

... And your body relaxes ... deeper and deeper ...

... Your gaze turns more and more ... inward ...

... And your body now releases all tensions ... let go ...

... And likewise, you can feel your muscles becoming ... looser ...

... You now also feel the ... relaxation ... of your tendons and ligaments ...

... You now also feel the ... relief ... of your joints ...

... Perception and attention work ... excellently in trance ...

... You yourself direct your attention to ... helpful words ...

... You recognize every helpful word ... exactly ...

... And you trust ... the helpful words ...

... and likewise ... you trust ... also in a deep relaxation of your body ...

... It is easy for you ... to concentrate on your body and its functions ...

... Therefore, you feel your breath ... very well ... and can feel every breath exactly ...

... You count the next five breaths ... {one breath pause} ...

... And all hardenings of your body are ... dissolved ...

... Feelings of pressure and pain are now significantly reduced ...

... You feel ... your body, and you feel your surroundings ...

... You can perceive the external and also ... the internal ...

... and your body reaches an ever deeper state ... of peace ...

... and a feeling of well-being spreads ... ...

... Feelings of pressure and pain go away, dissolve ...

... You trust ... in a truly deep relaxation of your body ...

... All hardenings of your body are ... dissolved ...

... Feelings of pressure and pain are now significantly reduced ...

... Your body reaches an ever deeper state ... of peace ...

... A feeling of well-being spreads ... within you ...

... Feelings of pressure and pain dissolve ...

... You feel your body with all your ... mindfulness ...

... You can therefore feel the ... peace and recovery ...

... You also feel that you are truly deeply relaxed ...

... You feel that your body is more deeply relaxed than ever before ...

... and all muscles are ... now truly ... loose ...

... All hardenings and feelings of pressure have actually ... completely ... dissolved ...

... And your body finds healing recovery, strength, and vitality ...

... You feel ... that your body is more deeply relaxed than ever before ...

... and all muscles are ... now truly ... loose ...

... All hardenings and feelings of pressure have actually ... completely ... dissolved ...

... And your body finds healing recovery, strength, and vitality ...

All Titles in the Series

Volume 1: Smoking Cessation
Volume 2: Anxiety and Restlessness
Volume 3: Burnout
Volume 4: Reducing Overweight
Volume 5: Coping with the Past
Volume 6: Suicidal Thoughts and Attempts
Volume 7: Psycho-Oncology
Volume 8: Obsessions and Tics
Volume 9: Self-Confidence and Decision-Making
Volume 10: Grief Work
Volume 11: Psychosomatics
Volume 12: Chronic Pain
Volume 13: Depressive Thoughts
Volume 14: Panic Attacks
Volume 15: Domestic Violence, Victim Support
Volume 16: Post-Traumatic Stress
Volume 17: Exam Anxiety and Stage Fright
Volume 18: Anti-Violence Training, Offender Support
Volume 19: Addiction Tendencies
Volume 20: Social Phobia and Fear of Contact
Volume 21: Nail Biting
Volume 22: Self-Awareness and Self-Love
Volume 23: Teeth Grinding and Night Clenching
Volume 24: Feelings of Guilt
Volume 25: Fear in Crowds
Volume 26: Fear of Flying, Aviophobia
Volume 27: Fear in Enclosed Spaces, Claustrophobia
Volume 28: Tinnitus, Ear Noises
Volume 29: Fear of Heights
Volume 30: Neurodermatitis

Volume 31: Finding Inner Balance
Volume 32: Overcoming Loneliness
Volume 33: Fear of Illness, Hypochondria
Volume 34: Anticipatory Anxiety, Fear of Fear
Volume 35: Jealousy in Relationships
Volume 36: Driving Anxiety
Volume 37: New Start after Separation
Volume 38: Fear of Injections
Volume 39: Heart Anxiety Neurosis
Volume 40: Overcoming Resentment and Anger
Volume 41: Resolving Blockages and Positive Thinking
Volume 42: Stress Reduction, Stress Management
Volume 43: Body Relaxation
Volume 44: Deep Relaxation
Volume 45: Fear of the Dark
Volume 46: Falling Asleep and Staying Asleep
Volume 47: Compulsive Buying
Volume 48: Restless Legs Syndrome
Volume 49: Bulimia
Volume 50: Anorexia
Volume 51: Overcoming Nightmares
Volume 52: Imagined Deformity
Volume 53: Overcoming Distrust, Finding Trust
Volume 54: Processing Failures
Volume 55: Humiliation, Emotional Hurt
Volume 56: Distressing Compassion, Vicarious Suffering
Volume 57: Self-Forgiveness
Volume 58: Self-Awareness, Self-Confidence
Volume 59: Saying No
Volume 60: Assertiveness
Volume 61: Setting Boundaries and Self-Assertion
Volume 62: Decision-Making Ability

Volume 63: Success Orientation
Volume 64: Ruminating, Circular Thinking
Volume 65: Accepting Pregnancy
Volume 66: Birth Preparation
Volume 67: Spiritual Opening
Volume 68: Joy of Life and Inner Lightness
Volume 69: Patience and Inner Peace
Volume 70: Fibromyalgia and Rheumatism
Volume 71: Irritable Bowel Syndrome, Crohn's Disease
Volume 72: Fear of Nausea, Emetophobia
Volume 73: Stuttering and Cluttering, Speech Flow Disorders
Volume 74: Concentration and Knowledge Anchoring
Volume 75: Vitality and Spontaneity
Volume 76: Searching for Meaning and Finding Goals
Volume 77: Life Crises, Life Events
Volume 78: Workaholism, Goal Obsession
Volume 79: Helper Syndrome, Helpless Helpers
Volume 80: Medication Abuse
Volume 81: Gambling Addiction
Volume 82: Internet Addiction, Smartphone Addiction
Volume 83: Hoarding Disorder, Compulsive Collecting
Volume 84: Conspiracy Thoughts, Overvalued Ideas
Volume 85: Fear of Operations and Treatments
Volume 86: Fear of Aging
Volume 87: Travel Anxiety
Volume 88: Anxiety When Urinating, Paruresis
Volume 89: Fear of Intimacy and Togetherness
Volume 90: Fear of Blushing
Volume 91: Coming Out in Homosexuality
Volume 92: Charisma Training
Volume 93: Migraines and Chronic Headaches
Volume 94: Overcoming Allergies, Bronchial Asthma

Volume 95: Normalizing Blood Pressure
Volume 96: Compulsive Perfectionism
Volume 97: Sports Hypnosis, Motivation
Volume 98: Sports Hypnosis, Performance Enhancement
Volume 99: Determination and Focus
Volume 100: Encountering the Inner Child
Volume 101: Cravings, Binge Eating
Volume 102: Stimulating Metabolism
Volume 103: Bipolar Mood Swings
Volume 104: Borderline, Identity Crises
Volume 105: Hypomania, Euphoria, Mania
Volume 106: Restlessness, Agitation
Volume 107: Nervous Breakdown
Volume 108: Adjustment Disorders
Volume 109: Self-Alienation, Depersonalization
Volume 110: Ending Self-Pity
Volume 111: Primary Gain of Illness
Volume 112: Secondary Gain of Illness
Volume 113: Bullying, Victim Support
Volume 114: Letting Go of Envy and Jealousy
Volume 115: Fear of Spiders, Arachnophobia
Volume 116: Fear of Dogs or Cats
Volume 117: Fear of Strangers, Xenophobia
Volume 118: Excessive Worries, Generalized Anxiety
Volume 119: Strengthening Sense of Responsibility
Volume 120: Unrequited Love, Heartache
Volume 121: Work-Life Balance
Volume 122: Letting Go of Unattainable Goals
Volume 123: Allowing and Accepting Help
Volume 124: Letting Go of Adult Children
Volume 125: Tourette Syndrome
Volume 126: Life Changes and New Starts

Volume 127: Accepting Life in a Wheelchair
Volume 128: Understanding and Overcoming Homesickness
Volume 129: Understanding and Overcoming Wanderlust
Volume 130: Dizziness, Meniere's Disease
Volume 131: Overcoming Aggression
Volume 132: Cutting and Self-Harm
Volume 133: Hair Pulling, Trichotillomania
Volume 134: Postpartum Depression
Volume 135: For Relatives of Dementia Patients
Volume 136: Self-Harm, Artificial Disorders
Volume 137: Activating Self-Healing Powers
Volume 138: Preventing Depression Relapse
Volume 139: Reactive Psychoses, Follow-Up
Volume 140: Obsessive Thoughts and Impulses
Volume 141: Compulsive Checking
Volume 142: Compulsive Counting, Symmetry Obsession
Volume 143: Compulsive Washing, Cleanliness Obsession
Volume 144: Compulsive Questioning
Volume 145: Dissociative Paralysis
Volume 146: Phantom Pain
Volume 147: Overcoming Complaining
Volume 148: Hay Fever, Pollen Allergy
Volume 149: Sexual Abuse, Victim Support
Volume 150: Standing Strong Against Sexism, #metoo
Volume 151: Binge Eating
Volume 152: Overcoming Thoughts of Revenge
Volume 153: Detachment from the Aggressor, Stockholm Syndrome
Volume 154: Courage to Separate
Volume 155: Chronic Fatigue, Exhaustion
Volume 156: Fear of the Future, Existential Anxiety
Volume 157: Excessive Worry About Children
Volume 158: Fear of Failure

Volume 159: Ending Distrust and Control
Volume 160: Dejection, Dysphoria
Volume 161: Boreout, Chronic Boredom
Volume 162: Bipolar Disorders, Relapse Prevention
Volume 163: Mania, Relapse Prevention
Volume 164: Nihilism, Feelings of Worthlessness
Volume 165: Thumb Sucking
Volume 166: Being Brave
Volume 167: Being Proud
Volume 168: Overcoming Shyness
Volume 169: Being Able to Delegate Responsibility
Volume 170: Being Able to Show Emotions
Volume 171: Letting Go of Guilt, Victim Support
Volume 172: Processing Guilt, Offender Support
Volume 173: Mood Swings, Cyclothymia
Volume 174: Lack of Drive, Vital Sadness
Volume 175: Hearing Voices with Reality Reference
Volume 176: Confident Communication
Volume 177: Standing Up for Oneself
Volume 178: Taking New Paths
Volume 179: Confident Job Application
Volume 180: No Longer Being Taken Advantage Of
Volume 181: End of Submissiveness
Volume 182: Depressive Numbness
Volume 183: Mood Drops, Affective Incontinence
Volume 184: Mood Instability
Volume 185: Somatoform Disorders
Volume 186: Stomach Ulcer, Psychosomatic
Volume 187: Accepting Amputation
Volume 188: Overcoming and Letting Go of Hatred
Volume 189: Ending Accusations
Volume 190: Allowing Tears, Being Able to Cry

Volume 191: Finding and Sorting Repressed Feelings
Volume 192: Somatoform Pain
Volume 193: Living Autonomously
Volume 194: Anhedonia, Joylessness
Volume 195: Persistent Sadness
Volume 196: Obesity, Food Addiction
Volume 197: Parents of Abused Children
Volume 198: Letting Go and Letting Be
Volume 199: Childhood Sexual Abuse
Volume 200: Fear of Loss

www.ingramcontent.com/pod-product-compliance
Lightning Source LLC
Chambersburg PA
CBHW030504220526
45464CB00006B/2656